Your Breasts:
An Owner's Manual

Your Breasts:
An Owner's Manual

Bob Hurwitz, M.D.
Marnell Jameson. M.A.

Forward by Bonnie Rush, R.T.

Writer's Showcase
presented by *Writer's Digest*
New York San Jose Lincoln Shanghai

Your Breasts: An Owner's Manual

Writer's Showcase
presented by *Writer's Digest*
an imprint of iUniverse.com, Inc.

For information address:
iUniverse.com, Inc.
5220 S 16th, Ste. 200
Lincoln, NE 68512
www.iuniverse.com

ISBN: 0-595-13279-0

Printed in the United States of America

Dedication

This book is dedicated to Betty Ford.

"Taking a new step, uttering a new word, is what people fear most."

Fyodor Dostoyevsky

Mrs. Ford gave a famous press conference in 1975, describing a breast lump. She made it possible for women to discuss breast care without fear, opening the door to hope and dignity.

CONTENTS

Forward

As a health educator, I found this book to demonstrate compassion for the needs of all women. It is a helpful resource for breast care and the many options now offered to deal with carcinoma of the breast. Thank you **both** for taking the time to write this valuable aid to all women and those that love them.

This would be a valuable addition to any woman's personal health library.

—*Bonnie Rush, R.T.*

INTRODUCTION

We have written this book as a helpful guide for American women to deal with the life-long risk of lumps, cysts and cancer. Others have written books from a surgeon's point of view. These are accurate and well-written but subconsciously contain a surgical bias, often leaving the reader the impression that she is destined for surgery of one kind or another.

This text is written from the point of view of a radiologist with 20 years experience in mammography. My co-author is a health reporter for the Los Angeles Times and a well-known advocate of women's issues.

Our goal is to answer questions we have heard time and time again in a frank but realistic fashion. Our discussions are **no** substitute for the opinions and recommendations of your own physician. The authors use the following convention: "I" refers to the radiologist and his personal experience. "We" refers to our common knowledge of women's issues and concerns.

One in eight American women will contract carcinoma of the breast in her lifetime. This book offers those women hope and compassion while arming them with empowering, even life-saving knowledge. Early detection and breast-conserving surgery are turning the tide.

This book is also about the team approach: you, your doctor, the radiologist and yes, the surgeon. Happy reading and good health!

CHAPTER 1
What Every Woman Needs To Know

• Understanding Your Breasts

The breasts are actually glands, although we don't usually think of them this way. Like other glands, they have a function: to prepare, store and dispense milk. If you could look inside your breast, you would see first a layer of fat and under this 15 to 20 lobes, comprised of smaller sections called lobules. Thin tubes called milk ducts connect the lobules to the lobes and carry milk to the nipple when a woman is breastfeeding.

• Who Gets Breast Cancer?

Although normal cells in the body divide at a steady pace, sometimes cells divide and multiply rapidly, forming a lump, or tumor. When the lump is comprised of normal looking cells, it is said to be benign, or non-cancerous. Those cells do not spread or invade surrounding tissue. If the physician determines that the lump is made of abnormal cells, it is malignant, or cancerous. That means some of the cells can invade surrounding tissue or break off and travel to other parts of the body.

When a woman discovers a lump in her breast, she always fears the worst. However, a diagnosis of cancer is not the worst that could happen. The worst is delaying a visit to your doctor out of fear.

The only sure way to know if a lump is cancerous is to have some tissue removed and examined under the microscope. Although four out of five breast lumps (80%) are benign, every breast lump must be evaluated for the possibility of cancer.

Breast cancer most frequently develops in the ducts, but it can also begin in the lobes or lobules. When confined to the ducts or lobules, the tumor is noninvasive. If it has spread to surrounding tissue or other parts of the body, the cancer is called invasive. If detected early, breast cancer can often be treated effectively.

• One in Eight

One in every eight women will develop breast cancer during her life-time. A woman's risk varies depending on age, rising sharply for those over 40.

Breast cancer is the most frequently diagnosed cancer in women in the United States. Each year, 180,000 American women are told they have breast cancer. Even though breast cancer is more common in older women, it also occurs in younger women, and even in a small number of men.

• Risk Factors

Every woman is at risk for breast cancer. Although some women are identified as having an increased risk of contracting breast cancer, more than 70% of cases occur in women who have no such identifiable factors.

The National Cancer Institute (NCI) has developed a breast cancer "risk tool" to help women assess their individual risk. Some experts caution that the program omits essential questions and may underestimate a woman's risk. Researchers say the tool can provide a reasonable esti-mate of a woman's chances of contracting breast cancer. It can be obtained by calling (800) 4-CANCER or by requesting it from the NCI website at cancertrials.nci.nih.gov. The Institute recommends that women go over their results with their doctor.

• Gene Testing

Medical technology has advanced dramatically in the past ten years, resulting in what some call a genetic revolution. Scientists can now examine genes within human cells and have identified specific genes linked to breast cancer. BRCA1 and BRCA2 genes control cell growth in breast tissue. Scientists estimate that alterations in the BRCA1 and

BRCA2 genes may be responsible for 5% to 10% of all the cases of breast cancer and for 25% of the cases in women under age 30. However, gene testing is recommended only in select cases since there are associated risks, limitations, and far-reaching consequences. A doctor and genetics counselor can help women determine whether or not gene testing is appropriate.

• Detecting Breast Lumps

Breast cancer can be treated most effectively if it is detected early, before it has grown or spread to other sites. The main ways to detect breast cancer are:

- mammography
- breast examination by a doctor or nurse
- breast self-examination
- ultrasound

• Mammograms

A mammogram is an x-ray of the breast. It can detect some cancers too small to be felt. Sometimes lumps that can be felt are not detected in a mammogram. Thus, women of all ages should have their breasts examined every year by a physician or trained health professional.

Much controversy has taken place about when it is best for women to begin getting regular mammograms. Based on recent research data, the National Cancer Institute now recommends that:

- All women in their forties or older who are at average risk for breast cancer should have screening mammograms every 1 to 2 years.

- All women who are at higher risk for breast cancer should ask their doctors about when and how often to schedule screening mammograms.

- **There are two kinds of mammography:**
  - *Screening* x-rays help radiologists look for breast changes in women who have no signs of breast cancer.
  - *Diagnostic* x-rays are for women who have unusual breast changes, such as a lump, pain, nipple thickening or discharge, changes in breast size or shape, or a suspicious screening mammogram.

Don't simply assume a mammogram is normal if the doctor's office doesn't contact you with results. Call and ask.

- **Clinical Breast Exam**

Since some cancers cannot be detected by mammography, women also must have periodic breast exams by a doctor or nurse. The provider will look at your breasts while you are sitting and while you are lying down.

- **The provider looks for:**
  - changes in the skin, such as dimpling, scaling or puckering
  - nipple discharge
  - change of size or shape in the breasts.

- **Breast Self Examination (BSE)**

Women should also begin examining their breasts monthly beginning at age 20. Every woman needs to become familiar with the way her breasts feel and look so that she can detect changes.

The best time to do BSE is 2-3 days after your menstrual period is finished. Here are general guidelines, but it's best to ask your healthcare provider to show you how to perform BSE to be sure you are doing it correctly.

1. First, look in the mirror and see if you detect any lumps or thickness, swelling, puckering, dimpling, redness, or soreness of the skin, as well as changes in nipple size or shape. Also squeeze the nipple to see if there is any discharge.

2. Stand upright with your right hand behind your head. Use the flats of your fingertips on your left hand to gently feel the breast, making small circles around the nipple, then make larger and larger circles as you work your way around the entire breast. Change and repeat the process on the other breast.

3. Do the same while lying down. Also feel the collarbone area and the armpit on each side.

• Ultrasound

Ultrasound sends high-frequency sound waves into the breast, creating patterns of echoes that are converted into an image of the breast's interior (a sonogram). Ultrasound helps radiologists evaluate those lumps that can be felt but are hard to see on a mammogram. Unlike mammography, ultrasound cannot detect small tumors.

• Magnetic Resonance Imaging (MRI)

The use of MRI for detecting breast cancer remains in the research stage. MRI uses a large magnet to surround the patient with radio frequencies and a computer to provide images. Its usefulness in identifying abnormal tissues is being actively studied.

CHAPTER 2
Breast Cancer: Three Steps Forward And One Step Back

The "War on Cancer" was declared in 1973. Small and effective improvements in detection and management suggest that this may be the longest war medical science has ever waged.

Three setbacks have occurred in mammography.

- First was in the 1970's, when a well-meaning statistician published a article suggesting that mammography caused more cancers than were detected. The medical community was outraged.

  The statistics were based on outmoded equipment and filming techniques no longer used. For ten years, the number of women willing to undergo mammography dropped dramatically. Meanwhile, manufacturers of mammography film and mammography equipment greatly improved their products. The term "low-dose" film-screen technique became a mantra that even today I sometimes see in reports across the nation.

- Second was in the 1980's when women became concerned that postmenopausal hormone replacement increased their risk of breast cancer. Because women taking hormone replacements noticed more breast pain ("mastalgia"), innocent cysts and other symptoms, they were led to believe this possibility.

  Once again, medical scientists were energized to action. Hormone replacements (HRT) were modified, combining both estrogens and progestins. The strength of each was slowly reduced to assure as few symptoms as possible. A non-estrogen synthetic compound (Evista®) is now available for those who will not accept estrogens of any type.

  Why were physicians concerned? Lack of hormone replacement dramatically increases the risk of coronary heart disease. Without estrogen, the risk of osteoporosis also dramatically increases. Hip fractures and vertebral compression fractures should not be tolerated in a modern society.

- Third came confusing media reports of "breakthroughs" in cancer detection and treatment. All reporters have access to the medical literature. Many articles describe new methods that are in preliminary research stages. Many require years of further study, testing, and independent verification. Still, it is tempting for reporters to take these journal articles out of context and describe a "breakthrough" that will make headlines (and a reporter's career). Almost weekly, a patient hands me an article of the latest news and asks, "Why don't American physicians know about this!"

CHAPTER 3
The Good News About Most Lumps

When a woman first learns she has a breast lump, her first reaction typically is panic. She needs to reassure herself that only one in five lumps is cancer: 80% of all breast lumps are not cancer. Some common benign breast changes that may feel like a lump include:

- *Fibrocystic condition:* Generalized breast lumpiness, this may become less obvious as women approach middle age and the milk-producing glandular tissue gives way to soft, fatty tissue.

- *Cyclic breast changes*: During the menstrual cycle, extra fluid often collects in the breasts. These can feel like lumps but usually go away by the end of the menstrual period.

- *Cysts:* These fluid-filled sacs often enlarge and become tender just before the menstrual period. Physicians usually treat them by observation or by fine needle aspiration.

- *Fibroadenomas*: These are solid, round tumors made up of benign tissue. They feel rubbery and can easily be moved around. Although they can sometimes be diagnosed with fine needle aspiration, most surgeons believe that it is a good idea to remove fibroadenomas to make sure they are benign.

- *Fat Necrosis*: Round, firm lumps sometimes form when fatty breast tissue becomes damaged and disintegrates. These typically occur in obese women with very large breasts.

- *Sclerosing adenosis*: These excessive growths of tissue in the breast's lobules can frequently cause breast pain. Without a biopsy, adenosis can be difficult to distinguish from cancer.

The only **certain** way to learn whether a breast lump or abnormality is cancerous is by having a biopsy.

In this procedure, a surgeon or radiologist removes some of the suspicious breast tissue, which a pathologist examines under a microscope.

There are different forms of biopsies. Though your doctor will determine which technique is best, here's a brief description of each:

- **Biopsy Methods**
  - *Excisional biopsy:* Generally used for lumps smaller than an inch in diameter, this method removes the entire suspicious area along with a small margin of normal tissue. This is usually performed in an outpatient department of a hospital with the use of local or general anesthesia.

  - *Incisional biopsy:* With this procedure, a surgeon slices a portion of the tumor for the pathologist to examine. This method is generally used for larger tumors and with general anesthesia.

  - *Fine needle aspiration:* Here, radiologists use a very thin needle and syringe to remove either fluid from the cyst or clusters of cells from a solid mass.

  - *Core needle biopsy:* This requires a somewhat larger needle with a special cutting edge to remove small cores of tissue. This technique may not work well for lumps that are hard or small.

  - *Localization biopsy:* In this technique, your doctor uses mammography to locate breast abnormalities detected by mammogram but not felt. The radiologist places a special needle to guide the biopsy.

  - *Stereotactic localization biopsy:* For harder to locate masses, radiologists use 3-D x-ray to guide the needle biopsy, with a computer plotting the exact position of the suspicious area.

- **The Pathologist**

The pathologist is a specialist who examines cells or tissues under a microscope, looking for abnormal cell shapes and unusual growth patterns. It is important to have a pathologist who is experienced in diagnosing breast cancer evaluate your biopsy slides.

When you get your biopsy results, I recommend you bring someone along to share the conversation with your doctor. If the diagnosis is cancer, you may be too upset to fully hear the important information your doctor will give you. Another set of eyes and ears can help. If all is well, you'll want someone to celebrate the news with.

If there is any question about the results of your biopsy, you may request that another pathologist also review your biopsy slides.

CHAPTER 4
When It's Cancer

Often when a woman hears the word "cancer", she completely blocks out anything the doctor says after that. No one can ever be truly prepared to hear that they have cancer.

No matter what the type of breast cancer, the effect on you depends on a number of factors, including your general health. One of the most important things you can do for yourself is to find others who have already gone through the anxiety of breast cancer to help you through the fear and worry. Now is **not** the time to withdraw.

Understanding the Stages of Breast Cancer

Breast cancer is usually diagnosed as falling into one of five stages. How your cancer is staged and your treatment choices depend on:

- How small or large your tumor is and where it is in your breast.
- If cancer is found in the lymph nodes in your armpit.
- If cancer is found in other parts of the body.

Here are some terms sometimes used to describe cancer:

- *Malignant*: the biopsy revealed the presence of cancer cells.
- *In situ or noninvasive*: a very early cancer or pre-cancer that has not spread beyond the breast.
- *Invasive:* cancer has spread to surrounding tissue in the breast and may have spread to the lymph nodes in the armpit or to other parts of the body.
- *Metastasized*: the cancer has spread to other parts of the body, such as the bones, lungs, liver or brain.

Staging Of Breast Cancer

Stage 0   Very early cancer or pre-invasive cancer that has not spread within or beyond the breast.
Stage 1   Tumor smaller than 2 cm (1 inch). No cancer is found in the lymph nodes in the armpit.
Stage 2   Tumor smaller than 2 cm (1 inch). Cancer is found in the lymph nodes in the armpit.   -or-   Tumor between 2 and 5cm(1 and 2 inches). Cancer may or may not be found in the lymph nodes in the armpit.   -or-   Tumor larger than 5cm (2 inches). Cancer is not found in the lymph nodes in the armpit.
Stage 3   Tumor smaller than 5cm (2inches) with cancer also in the lymph nodes that are stuck together.   -or-   Tumor larger than 5cm (2inches), or cancer is attached to others parts of the breast area including the chest wall, ribs, and muscles.   -or-   Inflammatory breast cancer. In this rare type of cancer, the skin of the breast is red and swollen.
Stage 4   Tumor has spread to other parts of the body, such as the bones, lungs, liver or brain.

Treatment of Carcinoma of the Breast

Prognosis

Once your doctor has determined the type and stage of the cancer, your chance of recovery will depend on many factors, including:

- The type and stage of cancer
- How fast the cancer is growing

- How much the breast cancer cells depend on female hormones for growth (as measured by hormone receptor tests). Tumors that are hormone-dependent can be treated by hormonal therapy.

- Your age and menopausal status

- Your general state of health.

Accepting your diagnosis at first will likely be difficult. Over time, that will change. Maintaining a positive attitude and seeking the support of friends and family will not only help you through this ordeal but will also contribute to your recovery.

Making Decisions

Treatments for breast cancer vary. Doctors used to perform biopsies and remove the breast all in the same operation. Thankfully, this rarely happens today. Women need time to absorb biopsy results, learn about their options, and perhaps get a second opinion.

Gone also are the days when doctors firmly tell patients what is best. Today, patients bear more and more responsibility for speaking with a variety of medical experts, gathering as much information as possible, and choosing from several treatment options.

Treatment Options

There are several options, and often more than one treatment is used.

- *Surgery:* taking out the cancer in an operation.

- *Radiation therapy:* using high-dose x-rays to kill cancer cells or keep them from dividing and growing.

- *Chemotherapy:* Using anticancer drugs to kill or stop the growth of cancer cells.

- *Hormonal therapy*: using hormones to stop cancer cells from growing.

- *Biological therapy (immunotherapy)*: using the immune system to fight cancer or to lessen the side effects that may be caused by some cancer treatments. Many biological therapies are being tested in clinical trials.

- *Bone marrow or stem cell transplants*: efficacy still being tested in clinical trials.

Types of Surgery

- *Lumpectomy*: a surgeon removes the breast cancer, a little normal breast tissue around the lump, and some lymph nodes under the arm. The surgeon's goal is to totally remove the cancer and to alter the breast as little as possible. Lumpectomy is usually followed by radiation therapy to destroy any remaining cancer cells.

- *Total mastectomy*: The surgeon removes the entire breast. Some lymph nodes under the arm may also be removed.

- *Partial mastectomy*: This surgery conserves as much of the breast as possible. Some breast tissue is removed, along with the lining over the chest muscles, and sometimes part of the muscle.

- *Modified radical mastectomy*: the surgeon removes the breast and some of the lymph nodes under the arm. Sometimes, parts of the chest wall muscle are removed.

- *Radical mastectomy*: The surgeon removes the breast, chest muscle, and all the lymph nodes under the arm. This was the standard operation for many years, but it is used now only when the cancer has spread to the chest muscle.

Radiation Therapy

High energy x-rays are used to destroy cancer cells that might still be present in the breast tissue. Doctors sometimes use radiation therapy following a lumpectomy or mastectomy, before or instead of surgery, and/or in conjunction with chemotherapy.

Possible problems: feeling more tired than usual, skin itchiness, redness, soreness, peeling, darkening, shininess, or decreased sensation. Radiation does not cause hair loss, vomiting, or diarrhea.

Chemotherapy

Even when a lump is small, cells may have broken off and spread outside the breast. Doctors can use chemotherapy to destroy them, using either a single drug or a combination of drugs.

The drugs are often injected into the bloodstream through an intravenous needle, but sometimes they are administered by pill. Treatment can range from two months to two years.

Possible problems: hair loss, loss of appetite, nausea, vomiting, diarrhea, constipation, fatigue, infections, bleeding, weight change, mouth sores, throat soreness, infertility, early menopause, weakening of heart, damage to ovaries, and secondary cancers (such as leukemia).

You can learn more about chemotherapy by contacting the NCI (1-800-4-cancer) and requesting the following booklets: "Helping Yourself During Chemotherapy," "Chemotherapy and You", and "Eating Hints for Cancer Patients."

Hormonal Therapy

If lab tests show that a tumor relies on your natural hormones to grow, any remaining cancer cells may continue to be stimulated by your body's hormones. Medications can prevent your body's hormones from reaching any remaining cancer cells.

Tamoxifen is one of the most common drugs used for hormonal therapy and is taken daily as a pill. Although benefits far outweigh risks, you should be aware that tamoxifen use increases risk of cancer of the uterus and, rarely, blood clots.

Possible problems: hot flashes, nausea, vaginal spotting, increased fertility. Less common side effects include depression, vaginal itching, bleeding, or discharge, loss of appetite, eye problems, headache, and weight gain.

CHAPTER 5
The Silicone Story

During the early 1960s, women underwent silicone injections to augment (increase) breast size. Carol Doda in San Francisco owned her own nightclub and quickly discovered that the more injections she had, the busier her club became. She retired, quite wealthy, and never had a problem with her enormous breasts.

Others were not so lucky. Free silicone produces lumpy changes in the breasts. Mammograms are simply of no value for detecting early cancer The silicone appears as numerous ovoid white lumps. Breast self-examination (BSE) is also useless. Fortunately, this technique was quickly abandoned in the United States.

Implants using a silicone-encased envelope became available in the late 1960s. During my plastic surgery rotation in medical school, these were passed around for inspection. There was uniform agreement that these felt natural and seemed to be the ideal replacement for the banned injection technique.

The several large manufacturers continued to refine the implants. They were well aware of the phenomenon of "bleeding", a slow microleak of the inner silicone through the silicone "envelope." The medical literature also did not show any concern or alarm. Silicone is used for many surgical devices. Every time you have your blood drawn for medical testing, the needle is lubricated with silicone for a less painful "stick". This remains the case even today.

In 1992, a small group of women with breast augmentation began to complain of rheumatoid and other autoimmune disorders. Dr. David Kessler, then director of the FDA (Food and Drug Administration), used his authority to halt breast augmentation.

I was amazed that so brilliant a physician as Dr. Kessler would take such a drastic step without first consulting others or insisting on data collection for the two million American women who had augmented breasts.

Whether it was political pressure or simply a fear that the medical community had placed these women in jeopardy will never be known.

Many of his other FDA decisions on approval of drugs and medical devices came under fire for his lack of leadership and inability to take the political heat of Washington politics. Dr. Kessler later returned to an academic post.

Dow-Corning, the largest manufacturer of implants, declared bankruptcy. A $4 billion trust fund was set up for any patient who could prove an illness due to breast implants. This company continues to provide information to patients and physicians on data that they collect. A Mayo Clinic report in the New England Journal of Medicine has disputed the whole matter. The Mayo found **no** increase in rheumatoid or other immune disorders in their augmented patients.

For several years, implants were made available only to a select group of test patients or those needing reconstruction after cancer surgery. The saline implant (with the same silicone envelope) was then approved. Today, more implants are placed than ever before.

Plastic surgeons first obtain a baseline mammogram to exclude any possibility of an unsuspected cancer. Radiologists like myself are pleased. Saline is less dense than silicone. Patients are less fearful. Even if a saline implant ruptures, the fluid is simply sterile salt water and of no health threat.

Should you have silicone implants removed? If you have no symptoms and remain pleased with the results, plastic surgeons advise leaving them in. On a happy note, I now have seen implants 25 years old. We will soon hit the 30-year mark in some patients.

CHAPTER 6
Men Have Breast Problems, Too!

Men have breast problems, including rare cases of cancer. The most common problem in men is gynecomastia. This is benign enlargement of one or both breasts and at any age. I often marvel at the surprised look on women's faces when they see a man waiting for his mammogram appointment. Though men are embarrassed, they're equally fearful.

Mammography in men is performed using the same technology as for women. Benign gynecomastia is either fatty or glandular. In either case, the images are definitive. The cause must then be discovered, usually always a medication that must then be eliminated.

Drugs Implicated as Causing Gynecomastia

Category	Drug
Hormones and steroids	Androgens and steroids, chorionic gonadotropin, estrogens and estrogen agonists.
Antiandrogens or inhibitors of androgen synthesis	Cyproterone, flutamide.
Antibiotics	Isoniazid, ketoconazole, metronidazole.
Antiulcer medications	Cimetidine, omeprazole, ranitidine.
Cancer chemotherapeutic agents	Numerous.

Cardiovascular drugs	Amiodarone, captopril, digitoxin, enalapril, methyldopa, nifedipine, reserpine, verapamil.
Psychoactive	Diazepam, halperidol, phenothiazines and tricyclic antidepressants.
Drugs of abuse	Alcohol, amphetamines, heroin and marijuana.
Other	Phenytoin and penicillamine.

One of our male employees complained of dramatic breast enlargement. The same fears came to him as to a woman with such a presentation: cancer and perhaps a premature death.

Mammography demonstrated benign gynecomastia. His wife had bought a freezer full of chicken at one of the local warehouse-type stores. Their daily chicken dinner exposed our patient to the hormones that some (but not all) chicken producers use to hasten growth of their "product."

Our employee discarded the frozen chicken and within months, his breasts returned to normal. This happy conclusion illustrates that mammography and a good medical history are not to be feared.

CHAPTER 7
The Five Golden Rules Of Every Good Radiologist

Radiologists, including myself, have learned important steps to build your confidence in our work. We want you back the next year for your annual mammogram, knowing that every possible step is being taken to make the study almost a calm and routine procedure.

Rule 1: Build and Maintain Rapport

I establish good rapport with you, my patient and your referring physician. Once established, I cherish it. Your concerns are important.

I strive to earn your confidence, respect and appreciation. Many physicians have said, "If I could just practice good medicine and not be burdened with the threat of malpractice affecting every decision or action…" I want my patients to feel confident that

- I am an expert
- I am aware of your concerns
- I care about your concerns
- I have given special attention to your concerns with additional views, sonography, and palpation
- I am available for your continuing or future concerns and that
- I want to see you again.

Rule 2: Careful Documentation

I document what I say, what your physician says, what I see, and what you might say while you are in my facility. My telephone communications are also carefully documented. Vague memories of comments, events, or specific instructions are no substitute for the written record.

Rule 3: I Note Your Concerns

I know and document your concerns and those of your referring physician. I listen to and seek information from patients and their referring doctors.

Rule 4: I Give Thorough Explanations

I know and document that the area of clinical concern has been adequately visualized and correlated with imaging findings. I try to explain what has clinically been noted. Is there any imaging finding to explain the clinical concern?

If there is no abnormality on your mammogram, both you and I know that the area has been well evaluated and everything appears normal. My recommendation will be: "Continue to examine yourself once a month and let your doctor know if there are changes or if you have any new concerns. I will be happy to check this at anytime. If there is no change, I would like to obtain another mammogram in a year".

Rule 5: When The Mammogram Is Normal

I do **not** document things that are not real. If an image shows something that's questionable, I provide appropriate information to see prove my explanation. Example: a fatty lobule that looks like a mass or cyst on ultrasound might look at first like a solid mass.

CHAPTER 8
The Sentinel Node Is Your Friend

We learned 20 years ago that tumors spread in an orderly fashion. Lymph node chains "drain" a tumor. They also protect us from infections. All of us have felt a groin or axillary lymph node that briefly is enlarged or tender.

For 15 years, I was an investigator in a trial of lymphoscintigraphy for staging of malignant melanoma. The protocol required injecting a minute amount of radioactive tracer around the melanoma. Images, using a special gamma camera, then proved where the lymphatics for that region drained. These are tiny, fluid-filled channels that course underneath the skin, leading to a lymph node "basin."

Surgeons verified this technique using a blue dye. I would mark the skin (in both men and women) where the "sentinel" or first lymph node should be excised. We knew then (and now) that this was a mapping procedure. The lymph node could well be free of any cancer cells and further lymph node resection was deemed unnecessary.

Workers at M.D. Anderson Hospital in Texas and the Moffett Cancer Center in Florida seized upon this concept and applied it to cancer of the breast. If the sentinel node in the axilla is negative for tumor, this dramatically improves your prognosis and minimizes the need to do extensive lymph node dissection.

We have now done hundreds of sentinel biopsies to stage breast cancer. Patients tell me that the previous and standard thorough lymph node dissection leaves them in greater pain and with more complications than the removal of the actual breast carcinoma.

Why has Sentinel Node Biopsy (SNB) proven so successful? The pathologist now can perform a more focused and extensive examination of the single node. Additional sections and immuno-histochemical analysis show an increased detection of micrometastases. Many studies quote between 25-50% more of these tiny foci of cancer when the single lymph node is more carefully examined.

When the Sentinel Node is proven free of tumor cells, there is little likelihood of spread of tumor to other nodes or to distant sites. This has been a dramatic step forward in care of breast cancer patients.

CHAPTER 9
I Heard It Through The Grapevine

As mandated by Federal Law, the revised MQSA (Mammography Quality Standards Act) of April 28,1999 requires that all radiology facilities call or write patients to notify them of their test results, whether normal or abnormal. Do not be alarmed by a call from a stranger. Even in the short time since MQSA was passed, I have discovered that women very much appreciate hearing news quickly. Your doctor may be out of town. Any number of things may delay your hearing good news or worrisome news.

Call-backs: About 10% of our screening mammograms require that women return for further evaluation. Usually, this requires additional views or even ultrasound to assure that the test was truly normal.

A call-back changes the screening mammogram into a diagnostic mammogram. This assures you that a radiologist will explain in layman's terms the results of the additional views.

On occasion, technologists see a problem on a screening mammogram that warrants immediate attention. In such cases, the radiologist will see a screening patient and accelerate the workup. This avoids the emotional stress of being called back. I always compliment the technologist (in the presence of the patient) on their initiative and compassion.

The practice of mammography is changing. Radiologists were used to calling the referring physician for permission to perform further tests. Today, however, radiologists now perform whatever further tests are necessary to draw a speedy conclusion to the examination. They are also required to tell you all results and what recommendations will be made, again something only your referring physician used to do. All has changed in the interest of better and faster medical care. This is a dramatic exception to the practice of medicine. In no other field of radiology has such a revolution taken place (nor is it likely to).

We've got your number!

The MQSA law further requires that radiologists categorize **every** single patient they see. The Bi-RADS ™ categories are as follows. Do not be alarmed by this development. It must be done whether findings are normal (negative) or worrisome.

Assessment Categories

0	Incomplete; need additional evaluation or prior films
1	Normal ("negative") mammogram
2	Benign findings
3	Probably benign findings; short interval follow-up suggested
4	Suspicious abnormality; biopsy should be considered
5	Highly suggestive of malignancy

CHAPTER 10
MQSA, FDA, ACR And BiRADS:
Alphabet Soup

Over the past 25 years, mammography has evolved as our most effective weapon in combating breast cancer. At the same time, mammography has become the medical examination most thoroughly scrutinized by the scientific community, the American public, and the media. Mammography is the most heavily regulated test in the history of medicine. Legislation dealing with mammography culminated in the passage of the Mammography Quality Standards Act (MQSA) in 1992, although the final version of the Act is only now taking effect.

In the early and mid-1980's the cost of a mammogram ranged from $50-$250. The average cost was well over $100. Most insurance companies adopted the policy of paying only for mammograms of patients who had symptoms or signs of breast cancer or those at "high risk." As a result, cost and access kept many asymptomatic women from getting screened.

In 1986 the ACS (American Cancer Society) with the support of the ACR (American College of Radiology) initiated the Breast Cancer Awareness Program. This provided low-cost mammograms throughout the country. Over the next three years, the average price of a mammogram decreased almost 50%.

As general awareness of mammography importance increased, mammography gradually became more accessible and affordable to more women. Access to mammography further improved when, in 1989, 20 national medical organizations endorsed consensus screening mammography guidelines. These guidelines recommended regular screening of all women 40 years of age and older.

The initial guidelines suggested annual mammography screening for women 50 and older and every year or two for women age 40-49. The American Cancer Society Guidelines now recommend annual intervals for all women over 40. For the first time, third party payers and clinicians alike could apply a widely accepted "uniform standard", paving the way for routine screening mammography.

The American College of Radiology (ACR) also responded with the establishment of the Mammography Accreditation Program (MAP). This program, developed at the urging of the American Cancer Society (ACS), comprised five parts: facility survey, phantom image evaluation, radiation dose measurement, clinical image evaluation, and processor performance. Although voluntary, the program quickly became the standard for quality mammography, with over 4800 facilities having applied for accreditation by early 1991. The ACR went on to publish Quality Control (QC) manuals for mammography in 1990, providing radiologists, radiologic technologists, and medical physicists with an easy to follow, cookbook-style approach to quality control.

PERSONNEL:

Interpreting Physicians must be licensed to practice medicine, and be certified by the American Board of Radiology (ABR) or receive three months of documented training in mammography interpretation. In addition, all interpreting physicians must:

- Acquire 60 hours of documented Continued Medical Education (CMEs) in mammography.

- Interpret mammograms from the examinations of 240 patients in a six month period.

- Continue to interpret at least 960 mammograms over a 24 month period. They must also obtain 15 hours of Continuing Medical Education in breast disease every three years.

Radiologic Technologists must be licensed by their states or certified by the American Registry of Radiologic Technologists (ARRT) and have 40 hours training in mammography. In addition, they must receive 15 Continuing Education Units (CEUs) in breast disease every three years.

Medical Physicists must be licensed or approved by the state or be certified by the American Board of Radiology or the American Board of Medical Physicists. In addition, they must receive 15 CEUs in breast disease every three years.

CHAPTER 11
Betty Ford: The Tide Turns

As a medical student at Johns Hopkins University, I was taught the dogma of William Halstead. He was a founder of the university and developed the radical mastectomy procedure. All of us were surprised that even as late as 1970, a woman would be anesthetized for a breast biopsy and not know if she would wake up with good news or a radical mastectomy.

In 1975, Betty Ford, First Lady of the United States, called a brief press conference. She announced that a lump had been found in her breast and that she was to undergo biopsy the next day at the National Naval Medical Center. The White House Press Corps was shocked. They had never heard the term "breast" mentioned in a room of men and women alike. They had never heard someone forthright enough to come forward and state "it might may be a cancer; we don't know yet."

Mrs. Ford promptly walked out to calmly host a State Dinner for the President of Italy. Her biopsy the next day was indeed positive for cancer, but she is living and well in retirement 25 years later in Rancho Mirage, California. While recovering from her surgery, she turned to Happy Rockefeller (wife of the Vice President) and encouraged Mrs. Rockefeller to have a screening mammogram. Incredibly, the mammogram was positive for bilateral cancers. Mrs. Rockefeller **also** remains in good health, living in quiet seclusion in upstate New York.

These two brave women made the word "breast" acceptable in public discourse. They also made it known to the world that screening mammograms find cancers early. Properly treated patients can indeed survive and live a long and active life. When Mrs. Ford and I first met in 1985 (she dedicated our breast care center), I was privileged to be in the presence of someone who conquered both cancer and a substance abuse problem. At a dedication luncheon, she spoke out on each of these matters not with personal concern, but only to give others hope.

Mrs. Ford and her daughter, Susan, conceived the concept of October as Breast Cancer Awareness Month. In 1999, the American College of Radiology expressed concern that uninsured women and residents of rural areas were not getting mammograms. October 15 was declared a day that such individuals should get a reduced price examination. This shall be a national voluntary policy.

CHAPTER 12
Who Was Susan G. Komen?

Following Mrs. Ford, many women came forward and declared their successful battle with carcinoma of the breast. The next was Nancy Reagan, another First Lady, also treated successfully and now retired to care for her ailing husband. Then came an incredibly brave woman, Susan G. Komen. She died of her disease at the age of 36.

Since then, Nancy Brinker, sister of Susan Komen, has been a tireless advocate of breast care. The Susan G. Komen Breast Cancer Foundation now has chapters nationwide. A network of volunteers staff an 800# help line (1-800-I'M AWARE). Ninety-eight Komen Race for the Cure® events are held each year throughout our country. The goal is to raise both funds and public awareness.

These runs include women's run/walk 5K events, mother/daughter and sister/sister teams. Co-ed and family runs also take place so that men (such as myself) have the honor of participating.

The Foundation makes an extra effort in Orange County, where I reside. We (for unknown reasons) have the highest incidence of breast cancer in the country. The Komen Race for the Cure® raises $1 million annually here in Orange County to assure that research, education and treatment for all can be funded.

Each year, Nancy Brinker comes up with even more ideas. More sponsors sign up, more families run/walk. Her goal is to prove that everyone is at risk: your mother, your wife, your friend, your daughter, your neighbor, your co-worker, yourself. In our area, another hero has emerged. Sandi Carter, herself a survivor of breast cancer, has won the 5K race seven of nine years, and has held our course record since 1993.

Corporate America has responded generously to the Komen Foundation. Lincoln/Mercury, Ford Motor Corporation, the Marriott Hotel Corporation and the Panasonic Industrial Corporation are among the sponsors. Also joining in are American Airlines, Johnson and Johnson, New Balance Shoes, the Tropicana Corporation, Pier 1 Imports and the NFL!

If Nancy Brinker has her way, her mission will "begin with a promise to her late sister and end with a cure."

CHAPTER 13
Lessons From Tillie

My first day of medical practice was a shock never to be forgotten. I was introduced to an inpatient, Tillie, who had metastatic carcinoma of the breast at age 18! She had only recently graduated high school. Despite her unusual name, she was the classic California blonde, tall and by all appearances, in good health.

Tillie fought the good fight, surviving another seven years. When visiting hours were over, nurses would have to chase out her dozens of boyfriends. Tillie was a friend to everyone, never complained, and accepted without hesitation any of the treatments that were then considered national protocols.

Tillie and I became friends through the years. I chatted with her about results of CT scans (computed tomography), chest x-rays, and ultrasound examinations. I would always express amazement that no matter what the treatment, she responded dramatically. Our private joke was that Tillie would get better even if her oncologist gave her shoe leather to chew on!

The lessons to be learned from this brave young woman were many and have not changed:

1. **Never** give up hope.

2. Medical therapy is constantly improving and worth the discomfort.

3. Family and friends are the best support group a patient can have.

4. Don't feel sorry for yourself. Feel sorry for those who just want to throw in the towel.

5. Doctors, nurses, and technologists are here to help. Tillie would effortlessly make friends. She knew everyone's name and had a smile that would melt anyone's heart.

6. Bad things happen to good people. Tillie was not the least concerned that she was only 18 when her seven-year journey of ups and downs began.

7. Tillie prepared her family and friends for the inevitable. She was the one in charge. A heroine, she shunned any publicity.

8. Tillie is probably looking down at us now, saying:

- **Doctors:** What's the latest good news on treatment?

- **Ladies:** Have you had your annual mammogram this year?

- **Families:** What are you worried about? The mind and body working together is a force to be reckoned with. If I could make such a statement in 1978, just think how far we have come since then!

CHAPTER 14
From The South Pole, With Love

One of the most incredible stories emerging from the war on cancer occurred in 1999 in the South Pole. Dr. Jerri Nielson was serving as the only physician for an American expedition at the Amundsen-Scott Station in Antarctica.

This 47-year-old woman discovered (on self-examination) a breast lump in June, 1999. Leaving Antarctica was out of the question. The South Pole is virtually cut off from the rest of the world between February and October. 24-hour darkness and sub-zero temperatures do not permit rescue aircraft to land.

Using the Internet, she received daily instructions. First there was an airdrop of a biopsy device on the ice. She then performed her own biopsy and diagnosed her own cancer. After relaying her findings via Internet to her physician, he decided to place her on chemotherapy at once. She administered the chemo herself!

When the Antarctic winter ended, a U.S. Air Force plane (equipped with skis for a brief ice landing) retrieved Dr. Nielson on October 16, 1999. The plane was on the ground only 22 minutes, taking off immediately in the face of temperatures of –60 degrees Fahrenheit and blowing wind and snow.

Dr.Nielson is now receiving appropriate therapy in the United States and has asked that further discussions of her medical condition be kept private.

During her four-month ordeal, she had a support group of 40 of her fellow researchers in Antarctica. She received frequent e-mail letters from physicians in the United States and remarkable support from students at her former high school in Dayton, Ohio.

The networking of physicians and friends kept up her spirits and proved that impressive strides have been made in cancer care, even in the face of the most incredible of circumstances.

CHAPTER 15
Villains And Heroes

Every story has to have villains and dashing heroes:

John Bailar, PhD. (villain). Two years before I began practice brought a startle to the medical community. Dr. Bailar, a brilliant statistician, wrote a famous article in the Annals of Internal Medicine. His article was titled: " Mammography: A Contrary View".

Seven pages of tortured statistical analysis led him to conclude: "the possibility is that mammography (due to radiation) takes almost as many lives as it saves." His conclusions were based on selected institutions where the procedure was performed poorly and with outdated equipment.

Dr. Bailar's "radiation scare" depressed mammography volume nationwide for nearly a decade. We will never know how many women lost a chance for an early cure.

The medical world was energized to combat this question: **better** equipment, **lower** radiation dose, and **better** training of radiologists. Rigorous national quality standards were published. By 1990, Dr.Bailar's claims were a distant memory. Even today, the lessons learned continue to annually improve both equipment and training programs in our Universities.

The Well-Meaning Reporter (Neither hero nor villain)

Nearly every week, a patient hands me an article about a new "breakthrough" that will replace mammography. These include articles quoting favorable early work in PET imaging, isotope imaging, digital mammography (image capture by computer), laser imaging and magnetic resonance scanning.

In each case, I politely explain that this is only promising research work. Mammography and breast ultrasound (if indicated) remain the standard of care in the nation.

In 1998, U.S. News and World Report published the very misleading article "No More Slam-o-Gram!" based on such research articles.

Gloria Frankel, M.D. (heroine), The late Dr. Frankel was a tireless advocate of mammography in the 1960s and 1970s. She taught physicians and women's groups that mammography finds cancer early and at a time when it is curable. The Kaiser System in California buckled under to Dr. Frankel's work and offered screening mammography to its patients.

The Health Insurance Plan of Greater New York (Hero). In 1963, the "HIP" began the world's first randomized and controlled prospective trial to determine if regular screening mammography (coupled with thorough physical examination) could reduce cancer deaths. After only seven years, cancer deaths dropped 30% in the screened group.

The American Cancer Society (Hero). Based on the astonishing results of the HIP study, a massive demonstration project began. 280,000 women enrolled in a study that became known as the BCDDP (Breast Cancer Detection Demonstration Project). The study reproduced the HIP results. The massive amount of data collected also revealed that there was much more work to be done to improve mammographic technology.

CHAPTER 16
Answers To The Most Commonly Asked Questions

Q: Are there good calcifications and bad calcifications?

A:Yes. Some calcifications in the breast are so classic that no further questions remain.

Good calcifications:

- A calcified fibroadenoma (a coarse lumpy calcification) This NEVER turns into cancer.
- "Milk of calcium": layering in a cyst.
- Oil cyst with thin calcified wall: A classic appearearance that NEVER turns into cancer.
- *Dermal calcifications*: These are in the skin, have clear centers, and are of no importance

Bad calcifications:

- Linear, branching, and tightly clustered calcifications. These are sometimes associated with a faint mass. These need removal either by core or open biopsy.

Indeterminate calcifications:

- Yes, sometimes we just can't tell! Magnification views and follow-up mammograms for as long as two years may be necessary. Lack of change is good news.

Q: I have calcifications. Should I stop taking my calcium supplements?

A: No!!! The breasts are metabolically active for life. These calcifications simply reflect the "Good calcifications" described above. Calcium supplements (with weight-bearing exercise) are the best protection you have against osteoporosis. More women get osteoporosis (with risk of fracture) than will ever get cancer of the breast.

Q: I have painful cysts. Should I restrict caffeine in my diet, take Vitamin E, or stop eating chocolate?

A: Research on these simple techniques is conflicting. I simply advise a trial of each method above for three months time. Then move to the next dietary step. If one or all three work for you, stay with it!

Q: My friends say to pick a woman radiologist/gynecologist/surgeon/oncologist. Are females better?

A: Surprisingly, not a single patient has ever objected to my being present, interpreting the mammogram or discussing all her questions. Certainly this is due to the relief a patient has that she can always ask for a second opinion from one of my five female colleagues.

Q: Should women only discuss with women physicians their concerns?

A: Again, the option is always there to choose. I am not offended by a request for a referral to a female colleague. With a female technologist acting as chaperone, women appear comfortable in asking me every possible question. The male/female barrier breaks down and the exchange of information appears the same as my female colleagues describe.

Appendix A

What You Can Do In The Fight Against Breast Cancer

- **Buy Postage Stamps**

The U.S. Post Office is committed to this cause. Beautiful 33-cent stamps featuring a woman's profile are for sale. Money is immediately sent to the American Cancer Society for research. Aware that the breakdown in its customers is 50/50 men and women, the Post Office also sells stamps promoting research for prostate cancer.

I purchase both of these stamps and try to use them in alternating order when corresponding to friends and family.

- **Join A Cause**

If Nancy Brinker, who started The Susan G. Komen Breast Cancer Foundation, can find a way to raise the nation's awareness, so can you.

    A. Register for one of the 98 nationwide Races for the Cure® events. Each event includes a simple one-mile run/walk so that an entire family can participate. Proceeds go toward research and education in each race community.

B. Women in distress about their health can call the Komen Foundation's national Toll-Free Hotline: 1-800-I'M AWARE.

C. For more information on this impressive and growing Foundation, visit their website: *www.breastcancerinfo.com*

• Buy Value-Added Clothing

If you wish a more discrete way of showing that you care, The Council of Fashion designers of America has a toll-free line naming which stores send a portion of their sales to the American Cancer Society for research and education. Call 1-888-771-2323 for more information.

• Get Informed

Your doctor is also a good resource for the latest information and counsel. This book cannot substitute for someone you know and trust. Reading this book is an excellent way to get informed.

• Write to the Authors

We welcome questions. Although the two of us are buried in e-mail each day, if you read something in this text and cannot get an understandable answer, e-mail us at: *mdlgl@mediaone.net*

We can't answer all of the mail we receive, but will try to answer those that require a prompt reply.

Appendix B
The Road To Recovery

If you are diagnosed with breast cancer, treatments are just the beginning of a lifetime journey. True, you are facing one of life's greatest challenges. Your return to day-to-day life may be prompt or slow, depending on your personality, condition, and many other factors. No matter how confident or despondent you feel, finding support can only help. Hundreds of people are eager to help if given the chance.

Your hospital may offer support groups or psychological counseling. Many other groups led by women who have survived breast cancer and now dedicate their lives to helping others. Here is a partial list of resources. These groups can likely put you in touch with many more.

Support Resources

- *The National Cancer Institute's (NCI) Cancer Information Service* provides specialists to answer questions, and help you find a breast cancer support group in your community: 1-800-4-CANCER.

- *National Alliance of Breast Cancer Organizations (NABCO)*: 1-888-80-NABCO

- *WIN- ABC (Women's Information Network Against Breast Cancer)* provides information and support to women with breast cancer. The Breast Buddy Care Program is a comprehensive program that provides information and support through decision-making, inpatient monitoring treatment, and recovery. A Breast Buddy volunteer is a survivor, extensively trained to educate and support breast cancer patients: (626) 332-2255.

- *Y-ME National Breast Cancer Organization* offers a national hotline, open door groups, early detection workshops and many local chapters. Through peer support programs, which include breast cancer patients talking with survivors and spouses of patients talking with spouses of survivors, Y-ME helps thousands of people each year who are concerned about or personally affected by breast cancer. 24 hour, toll free hotline: 1-800-221-2141 (English); 1-800-986-9505 (Spanish).

- *American Cancer Society*: 1-800-ACS-2345 (Check your phone book for the chapter nearest you.)

- *National Women's Health Resource Center* is the national clearing-house for the women's health information. If you become a member, the organization will research specific women's health topics for you: (203) 537-1015.

- *Public Health Service's Office of Women's Health: National Women's Health Information Center* provides comprehensive information and links to other resources and publications: 800-994-WOMAN

Steps to Take

Whether your risk of breast cancer is average or higher, here are steps you can take:

- Get regular breast exams by a doctor or a nurse and ask your doctor when you should begin getting regular mammograms.

- Exercise and eat a balanced diet that provides a good variety of nutrients and plenty of fiber. Limit dietary fat and alcohol.

- Consult your doctor about your personal situation and carefully weigh any potential risks against the benefits when making decisions about hormone-containing drugs.

APPENDIX C
Help from The Internet

More men and women are seeking health information from the Internet then from most any other source. The table below lists the most commonly visited sites during 1999.

Top sites for consumer healthcare information	
Drkoop.com	1.5 million
www.nih.gov	1.2 million
thriveonline.com	778,000
betterhealth.com	724,000
intllihealth.com	686,000
mayohealth.com	650,000
mediconsult.com	646,000
onhealth.com	618,000
ama-assn.org	339,000
ahn.com	318,000
medscape.com	281,000

healthanswers.com	271,000
healthcentral.com	236,000
healthy.net	198,000
webmd.com	188,000
americasdoctor.com	156,000
druginfonet.com	139,000
healthfinder.gov	114,000
medicinenet.com	98,000

Sources: Media Matrix and USA Today

We often worry that the so-called "dot.com" sites might have hidden agendas. There is frequent advertising. The information given may be biased to please a sponsor. Usually, however, the information provided is quite accurate.

We prefer Web Sites that end in .org, .net, .gov, or .edu These are non-profit entities that give unbiased information and accept **no** advertising.

Here are our favorite eleven Internet sites (the list grows daily).

www.nih.gov	*A brilliant site:* Skip directly to the "NIH Search Engine" to look up any questions about breast disorders.
mayohealth.org	*Constantly updated:* Skip directly to either the Cancer Center or Women's Center. This site is interactive
ama-assn.org	Frequently overwhelmed site.

healthy.net	*Skip to "Site Search":* Healthy.net balances conventional and alternative medical therapy.
healthfinder.gov	*Our favorite site:* Your tax dollar at work and well organized. The search engine is right at the top.
www.breastcancerfund.org	*A visually beautiful site:* The organizers are activists who take strong positions on the day's news.
www.nabco.org	A network of organizations dealing with all aspects of breast disorders.
www.2chicks.org	The "Chick Chat" section is lively and frequently contains information women are reluctant to discuss with their physicians
www.breastcancerinfo.com	*The Web Site for the Susan G. Komen Foundation:* Accurate headline news makes this the fastest of all the Internet sites
www.4women.org	*Web Site for The National Women's Health Information Center:* Updated daily by the U.S. Department of Health and Human Services.
cancertrials.nci.nih.gov	*The Web Site for the National Cancer Institute:* Everything you ever wanted to know about clinical trials, including medications to prevent breast cancer in high risk patients.

Notes: #1
My Medical History (Part I)

1. Date and place of last mammogram:

2. Physicians all reports should go to:

3. Any biopsies in the past?:

4. When and which breast?:

5. Any current breast complaints?:

6. Hormonal replacement therapy (now or in the past)?:

7. Any family history of breast carcinoma?:

8. Maternal side? Paternal side?:

9. Do I now have or previously have had augmented breasts?:

10. Do I practice monthly breast self-examination?:

NOTES: #2
My Medical History (Part II)

1. Do I keep copies of previous mammogram reports?:

2. Other medical illnesses in the past?:

3. Medications other than hormone replacement?:

4. Physicians and Medical Institutions I have seen in the past:

5. Other cancers I or my family have had in the past:

6. Are my breasts painful during the menstrual cycle?

7. Have I ever been told to restrict caffeinated beverages and chocolate or take Vitamin E?

NOTES: #3

My Duty Whenever I Schedule a Mammogram

1. Provide a signed release for reports and films from any other facility at which I have had a mammogram in the past.

2. Provide a written prescription from my doctor/health care provider.

3. Fill out the "intake" questionnaire fully and honestly. These questions are for **my** benefit. The X-rays will be tailored for any problems I have now or in the past.

4. Understand the difference between Screening and Diagnostic Mammograms.

NOTES: #4
The Responsibility of the Mammography Facility

1. **All** Radiologists have fulfilled their continuing education requirements (CME's)

2. **All** Technologists have fulfilled their continuing education requirements (CEU's)

3. **All** Mammography equipment has passed its annual FDA (Food and Drug Administration) inspection.

NOTES: #5
What Signs Should be Posted at Every Mammography Facility?

1. The "Patient's Bill of Rights".

2. The FDA/MQSA/ACR Accreditation Sign.

3. The Standard "Are You Now or Could You Be Pregnant?" Sign.

NOTES: #6
I Saw It On Television!

1. Medical information on television is (in our opinion) the **last** place you want to look.

2. TV shows, documentaries and "exposés" are tilted to garner ratings and advertising revenue.

3. Your best sources for unbiased information remain your doctor and the Web sites listed in the three Appendices of this book

Notes: #7

No One Has Taught Me Breast Self-Examination (BSE)

1. Physicians and other health care providers are sometimes too busy to emphasize, teach and confirm that you are doing proper BSE.

2. BSE is discussed thoroughly in this book.

3. A Breast Self-Examination shower card is available at no charge from Saks Fifth Avenue by calling 1-888-771-2323.

NOTES: #8
Why Me?

1. *Patients tells us that it seems unfair that they have a breast lump, breast pain, or even carcinoma.*

2. *We answer that this Millennium has brought improved care. Breast conserving surgery, in-office biopsy, core biopsy and sentinel nodes are all major breakthrough in women's health.*

3. *Excellent books are available on "why bad things happen to good people."*

4. *All large hospitals have support groups for concerned women.*

5. *The three appendices of this book list toll-free numbers to call for help and advice.*

NOTES: #9
My Friends and Neighbors Say to File a Lawsuit

1. *Attorneys make bad physicians and vice-versa.*

2. *Cancer starts with a single abnormal cell. No test is perfect! Neither are your doctors!*

3. *We have observed that no amount of money can compensate for the stress of breast cancer.*

4. *4-10% of breast cancers are missed, even by the nation's leading experts.*

5. *95% of medical malpractice suits end up in settlement. Your doctor, radiologist and surgeon carry malpractice insurance just for that reason. Medical bills for treatment can be paid from this insurance.*

6. *The stress of a lawsuit is shared by all parties. Cancer patients recover more quickly when they spend more time with their doctors and less time in an attorney's office.*

My Notes: This Book and
My Future Care